Super
tip

Supermodel tips

beauty and style secrets
from the world's top models

CARLY HOBBS

EBURY
PRESS

1 3 5 7 9 10 8 6 4 2

Ebury Press, an imprint of Ebury Publishing
20 Vauxhall Bridge Road
London SW1V 2SA

Ebury Press is part of the Penguin Random House
group of companies whose addresses can be found
at global.penguinrandomhouse.com

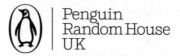

First published by Ebury Press in 2016

www.eburypublishing.co.uk

A CIP catalogue record for this book
is available from the British Library

ISBN 9781785033070

Printed and bound in Great Britain by Clays Ltd, St Ives PLC

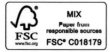

'Real beauty is everywhere and you just need to be open to the opportunity of seeing it with your heart and soul. There are so many things that make a woman beautiful. Confidence, integrity and talent are just some of them.'

Cara Delevingne

Contents

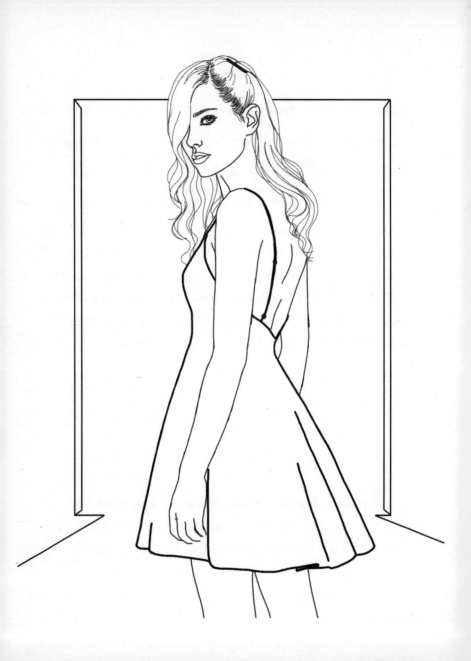

Supermodels. Beautiful, confident, powerful. Incredible skin, stunning make-up, beyond hot hair, lean bodies and a kick-ass kinda attitude. It looks like the most glamorous of lives. And of course it can be, but there is also a lot of hard work that goes on behind the scenes. Although many supermodels have a squad of facialists, make-up artists and hair stylists, and are treated to the flattering skills of retouchers who know how to work Photoshop to their advantage, they also put the effort in.

Between dashing from shows to shoots to interviews and red carpet events they pay particular attention to what they eat and drink, beautifying their bodies from the inside out. They work out regularly, honing and toning every six-feet-something-inch of their figures. They make sure they take time out, do things that make them happy and every now and then, on the rare chance they get a moment to pause, they take it all in, being mindful of what they have achieved, what they've experienced and what's yet to come.

Life as a model can be tough. They are constantly judged on their looks, style and attitude, once just by editors and casting directors, now by the world thanks to the explosion of social media as their lives are tracked on Twitter, Instagram, YouTube and Snapchat. But it's also incredible, as these are the women squeezing every beautiful moment out of their crazy, hectic and fun lives. And making it look extra pretty while they're at it. That's why we want in.

Anyone can take on the tips, tricks and mantras of the world's top models. From taking selfies to nailing your skincare routine and getting your eating, not to mention exercise schedule, in order. By taking on their ethos, we can enhance our everyday lives. That kick-ass attitude comes with practice, dedication and deciding to look at life a little differently, creating that level of happiness that makes everyone look like the most beautiful versions of themselves. And here, Kate, Karlie, Cara and co show you how to get started. They reveal how you can get their looks, bodies and attitudes, with a whole lot of fun as well as practicalities thrown in. And the best bit? It's simple to get started. Each quote inspires, and you can style out every tip away from the backstage area and studio. Ready, set, pout…

Make-up

'I really like the philosophy of "less is more". I want to see my skin, and see my own features. I want to use products to enhance my features, but I don't want to change or hide them.'

Christy Turlington

A fresh, glowy complexion that gleams rather than sheens is the epitome of supermodel skin, and you can achieve it by adding just one extra layer of make-up between your moisturiser and foundation. Work an illuminating cream across the cheeks, temples, forehead and jawline before buffing over your base using the same brushes. The end result? A seamless, 3D, flawless finish that's seen on catwalks all over the world.

Want model-perfect eyeliner in a flash?
Take the three-step approach. Supermodels
and fashionistas swear by its ease and finish.
Simply line the lid all the way along at the root
of the upper lashes, dot where you want your
flick to finish, then join up the two.

'If you're wearing smoky eye make-up, a little beige or gold pencil on the inner eye corners will open up the area, but you only want to do it if the shadow is really dark.'

Gisele Bündchen

Powder, translucent or matched to your skin tone, is a supermodel's BFF. Not only will it stop shine on that pesky T-zone area, but it is the ultimate backstage secret to stopping that eyeshadow-and-eyeliner-halfway-through-the-day-crease. The eyelid is the oiliest part of the face, so the powder absorbs this allowing your eye make-up to stay perfect all day long.

Dip cotton buds in micellar water and keep them to hand when perfecting liner and lippy; the cleanser swipes and lifts away mistakes rather than smudging.

A classic red lip works on *every* supermodel. And us. Go for an orangey red if you have a warm complexion, and a pinky, ruby hue if you own a cooler skin tone.

Get a perfect pout the same way the top models do – by buffing dead skin and flakiness from their lips with a secret blend of olive oil and brown sugar. Tasty and effective.

'If in doubt put a lip on.'

Jourdan Dunn

Well-groomed, full brows shape your face like nothing else, adding definition to give the whole face more structure as well as making us appear more awake. And behind the scenes they are being filled in with pencils and gels. Whatever your product preference, draw in individual hairs where yours are lacking.

Worried about smudging a statement lip? Press translucent powder into the pout to stop it budging or the colour escaping while making it last a whole lot longer. Top make-up artists do this for models on photoshoots all the time!

'A lipstick is an accessory.
It's the finishing touch on any
look. Whenever I wear deep red,
I feel mysterious and flirty.'

Joan Smalls

Models love spritzing fixing sprays over their faces – they keep all that make-up hard work in place. But did you know they also spray them on before their base? The extra layer gives the products something to hold onto, so you'll get less slip later on.

Mascara alert! Models or the pro MUAs on their teams apply mascara to the bottom lashes then do the top ones. Traditionally it's the other way round. However, when you do bottom lashes you tend to open the eyes wider, meaning anything already on those upper lashes gets transferred to the eyelids. Therefore doing the lower ones first stops this from happening.

Not in a mascara kind of mood? You can still add definition, backstage style, by rubbing a little Vaseline over your fingertips, then carefully smoothing onto lashes. Pretty. And zero smudging issues.

'I don't wear make-up every day, but I love to wear it for special occasions and mark the transition from day to night.'

Cara Delevingne

Want to recreate an avant garde beauty look? Inspired by the catwalk craziness of throwing glitter, shimmer and pigment all over the show? Ensure your artwork stays where you want it on your face by using cling film! Apply your base as usual, then before using sparkly products on eyes, pop little patches of cling film underneath. Top MUAs do this backstage as it catches all the pigment, then you can peel it off without making a mess after your look is complete.

Supers and their MUAs keep contouring subtle but effective by working taupe and matte brown powders and creams into the hollows of the cheeks to create flattering shadows. Pretend you're sucking a lemon if you're struggling to find the right place.

Want to define a jawline of supermodel proportions? Sweep a little contour cream – ideally in natural, earthy tones a few shades darker than your natural colour – along the sides of your jaw then blend until barely visible. Slim in 60 seconds.

'I always take my make-up religiously off at night. It doesn't matter how late of a night it is — or how intoxicated I might be — the make-up always comes off.'

Rosie Huntington-Whiteley

Models always highlight in a refined fashion.
Dust a sheeny product – pinky shell-like colours
for cool ladies, golden hues for warmer ones –
along the upper cheekbones. Don't take it further
than in line with your pupils though, else things
start to look sweaty rather than slick.

Want to pout it out on Instagram just like Cara, Karlie and Kate? Plump your lips the oh-so-natural way, by dotting a little liquid illuminator over the shape of the Cupid's bow. Pat in with your fingers until you can barely see it and use lippie as normal.

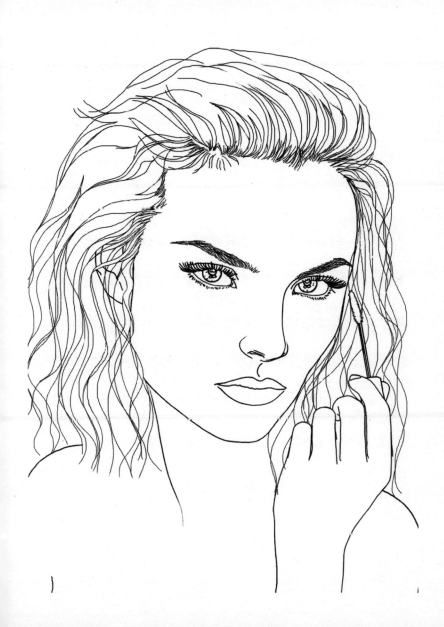

'Wherever I travel around the world, I always like to find cool little beauty products that are unique to each market but that aren't super expensive. They're treasures; when I bring them back to my sisters or friends it's more exciting than typical gifts.'

Karlie Kloss

Models have insanely hectic schedules. So they are always faking wide-awake eyes. You can too. Simply use a powder highlighter beneath the brow arch and right in the inner corners of the eyes and only apply mascara to the top lashes.

Beware product overload alert! Catwalk pros never use more make-up than they need, especially when it comes to base. Less is more. Using the back of your hand like a palette for your foundation, build up colour across your cheeks and buff it in with a second stipler brush.

It's model behaviour to add a little blush to any make-up look. Peachy corals are failsafe for everyone. Do a super-smile to find the apples of the cheeks then blend outwards from there.

'When I go to an event, I'll take a little container of loose powder and blotting papers... You really just need something to reduce shine. After I take the sweat and oil off my face with blotting paper, I'll use this tiny Shu Uemura brush to apply powder.'

Heidi Klum

Brushes. Wash them. Every single week Models have fresh, clean tools used on them at every job. You can use a brush a few times before washing, but always give them a clean with washing-up liquid diluted in water, then spray with an anti-bacterial cleaner. This eliminates product and bacteria build-up. It also means tools are effective rather than sluggish. Just remember to dry them properly.

Models can often be found using toothpaste to brighten their nails. Seriously. It removes that yellow tinge.

Short nails? File them into square, strong shapes. If they are longer, a rounded, more stiletto shape will look best.

'I'm cool to go make-up free, but usually to make myself feel better, I'll throw on a light foundation and some mascara.'

Kendall Jenner

Before layering on nail colours, give your talons a swipe with a cotton bud dipped in remover. It removes traces of dust and dirt so the varnish can sit smoothly.

Every good model's manicurist always has cotton buds dipped in remover to hand. Any spills or smudges can be quickly cleared up.

'Do a lip liner not to exactly line your lips, but to put it underneath just so it stays, and then if you want a super-super matte, you can put a translucent powder over the top.'

Georgia May Jagger

In a model-esque rush? No time to let your nails dry? Do one thin layer in a sheer shade, then run them under cool water to set the polish. It won't make them dry completely, so you still need to be careful, but it does reduce the chance of smudging.

Black mascara is a classic. It's bold and gives lashes a striking finish. However brown mascara is much more flattering, softer, cooler and less likely to cause an unintentional Panda-esque make-up look.

'Hold a credit card behind your lashes when you apply your mascara. If you press against the card you get a wide-eyed, curled effect without getting lots of product on your eyelid.'

Jourdan Dunn

No matter what show, what catwalk and what city, one thing is guaranteed backstage. Blending. From bases to eye colours, contours to cheeks models are having their make-up buffed to perfection. Always use a stiff brush to add product then a fluffy one to blend. It's the most model make-up thing you can do.

Fashion

'*Life is too short to always wear black.*'

Karlie Kloss

Just like Karlie says, black for life is boring. However, if your inner model still only wants to wear darks and neutrals, add the colours with shoes, a bag, a scarf or a piece of statement jewellery. Go on, try it, Rainbow Bright!

Whatever outfit you are wearing, imagine that there is a bunch of helium balloons tied to the top of your head on a tight piece of string, constantly making you hold your head high. Now keep your shoulders back and walk tall. That's model posture sorted.

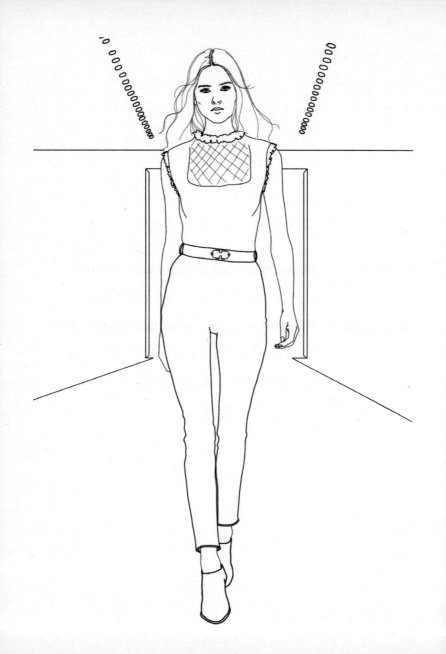

Models get to wear a host of clothes all the time, but you will actually find most are capsule wardrobe owners back home. Whenever they buy a new item it needs to work with current pieces to make at least three different outfits. Follow suit. Literally.

'Dress your attitude, not your age.'

Twiggy

Just because it suits your sister, friend, that model-a-like you saw strolling down the high street, it doesn't mean it will suit you. Stay true to yourself. When was the last time you saw Naomi and Kate wear the same thing? Exactly. Each to their own.

All models agree: nothing looks as good as confidence feels. Every item in your wardrobe should make you smile – be it the way it perfectly caresses your hips or because of a happy memory it takes you back to.

A little bit of skin goes a very long way and models rarely get it all out at once. Legs or décolletage. Arms or tummy. Operate the backstage rule of one in, one out.

Less isn't always more, especially when it comes to accessorizing with a supermodel attitude. Glam up any look by layering up necklaces. Mix different lengths, textures and colours, blending in a few of the same every now and then for cool consistency that will pull the whole thing together.

'I store my beauty products in a toiletries bag that's waterproof, so if there's a spill, my clothes are safe.'

Arizona Muse

Want to know three items ALL supers have in their wardrobe? A good fitting pair of jeans, a slightly battered leather jacket and a crisp white shirt. Classic, effortless, flattering.

Even when she's six feet tall you will never see a catwalk regular – backstage, on the runway or otherwise – sporting a trouser leg that is just that little bit too short. It's a fashion nightmare, so always try on trousers with the highest shoes you'll ever wear them with.

If it's not flattering don't buy it. Simple.
Top models never waste time styling out
items that don't work for them.

Get your boobs measured regularly! Everyone's breast size can go up and down. Ensure they're fitted properly in a range of amazing bras and every outfit will sit just right.

Your waist is The One when it comes to dressing like a supermodel: cinch it in, draw attention to it, wrap it in a belt, style out a thicker, tighter waist band … and always pose with your hands on it, not your hips!

'As a model for more than 25 years, I've had to wear lots of revealing outfits that can be difficult to manoeuvre. But sometimes wardrobe malfunctions happen. If you do have one, don't overreact and attract more attention to yourself. Gracefully put yourself back together, or get someone to help you if you can't do it on your own in an elegant and discreet way. We've all been there!'

Naomi Campbell

High heels are hot. Fact. They slim silhouettes and make legs look lean. BUT. They are tricksy to walk in, as anyone who has taken a tumble on the runway knows. So practice. Wear your highest heels around the house, strut to Beyoncé while hoovering, dance in the kitchen … as all good models know, practice makes perfect.

Top models learn from the stylists who dress them for shoots and shows, and always have a stash of safety pins and a mini sewing kit about their person. Handy for splits, rips and general fashion emergencies.

Skincare

'Keeping your skin healthy is the most important thing. Just having that natural glow is better than what any make-up can do for you.'

Gigi Hadid

Water. You know the model drill. Drink at least eight glasses a day for fresh skin and top energy levels. Chill bottles of tap water in the fridge, adding slices of cucumber and lemon to mix things up.

Top models love stashing their face creams in the fridge when on location to cool their faces post-shoot! Do the same on your holidays, or even when the weather is warm at home.

Spots in general should be left alone; ask any model or backstage beautifier. However, if they are white and ready to pop you can squeeze without scarring. You just need to do it in a super-clever and, most importantly, clean way. Dip two cotton buds into antiseptic, then push them together, against the spot. Use a third bud to swipe over the aftermath. Then: Do. Not. Touch.

'I like misting my face with rosewater every morning. It's so refreshing! It's moisturising and great for the winter when my skin gets really dry.'

Karlie Kloss

Models always fly minus their make-up, even in first class. It lets skin breathe and means you can apply hydrating oils and moisturisers mid-flight to keep your face as supple as possible. You can slick on some base, blush and mascara to face the paps – or friends and family! – upon landing.

After an alternative make-up remover? Every model's trusty go-to coconut oil will swipe away grime, product and leave skin beyond hydrated!

Catwalk regulars know that a golden glow gives them body confidence when doing their thing. Ensure your facial faux tan is even by having a cool shower prior to application to encourage pores to close, so the skin surface is as smooth as possible.

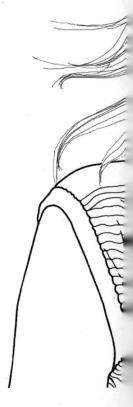

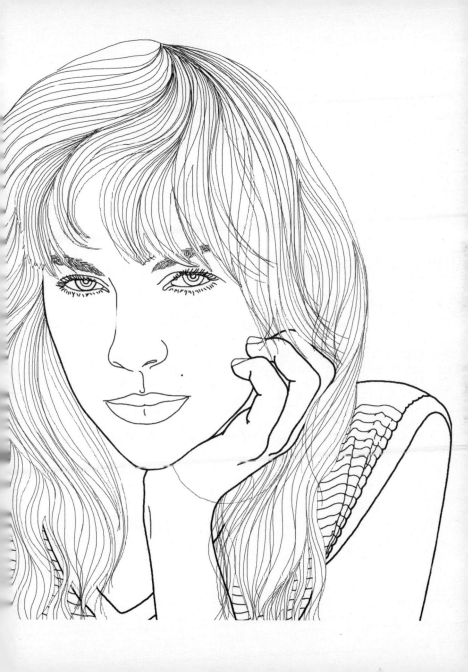

The most delicate area of skin is under the eyes: it's paper thin and shows the first signs of ageing. Keep wrinkles and sagging away by using a specialist eye cream and pitter-pattering it around the orbital bone with your fingertips. A top model beautician tip, this rain drop application limits movement while also boosting blood flow to the area, meaning increased skin cell turnover.

Even models take a day, or three, off make-up when not working. Let your skin breathe but don't forget to use a moisturiser with an SPF, which you do every day even under make-up, right?
Of course you do.

Cleansing once just isn't enough. Try using your usual face wash, then try a cream or micellar water cleanser with a cotton pad straight afterwards. You'll find another level of grime and make-up still comes off.

'Get bikini ready by scrub, scrub, scrubbing. I dry brush, wet brush, use scrubs in the shower — I'll try any kind of scrub. It's a terrific way to refresh, detoxify and soften the skin.'

Elle Macpherson

Your daily supermodel skincare routine should go like this: Every morning start with a double cleanse. Work on a serum or oil, which will go deeper than a cream to nourish every layer of skin cells. Pat on an eye cream. Smooth on a day-time specific moisturiser. Then before bed use both cleansers again, before generously applying a night cream, which will be richer and works its repairing magic as you sleep.

Face wipes are rarely seen backstage. More often than not top MUAs will prep cotton pads with cleansers so that models can quickly take off their look after walking in a show. Why? Face wipes can be harsh to skin and can also spread bacteria. To avoid flare-ups and blemishes only use as a last resort. Model note: they're better than leaving make-up on!

'I love coconut oil, so if I come home at night feeling all dry and like a fossil I'll put my hand in a jar of coconut oil and just mush it over my face.'

Suki Waterhouse

Make sure you massage in your moisturiser. Work it on with the tips of your fingers in circular motions. You can do this with cleansers too to boost circulation.

'I've always loved beauty products, but I didn't really get into skincare until my thirties. I've worn sunscreen every day since I turned 33. My whole routine changed, actually. I do all of those lotions and potions, toner, exfoliation, masks, all of it. I really like Vitamin A and C serums and oil-free moisturisers. None of it takes me too long, and I like the time I spend doing it.'

Linda Evangelista

What do all models have in common? They all exfoliate, around twice a week, more if their faces need it. Why do they carry out this top tip? It gently buffs away dead skin cells, which do build up, bearing in mind a skin cell cycle is about six weeks. They don't have to be grainy – you can exfoliate with fruit-enzyme packed products. Alternatively, make your own by mixing dried oats with water and buffing all over the face before rinising.

Supers love a workout... of the face variety. Opening and closing the mouth in a dramatic fashion as you say 'oh, ah, oh, ah' for five minutes every day tones up the skin and jawline while adding plumpness thanks to increased blood flow.

'You can get away with a late night with a tan — it covers a multitude of sins.'

Kate Moss

'If you have puffy eyes, a great trick is using really thick Greek yogurt with a little bit of honey and putting it under your eyes.'

Lily Aldridge

Models' handbags are packed with showbiz invites, bottles of water and little packets of almonds! These nuts are the snack equivalents of a facial as they are all about Vitamin E – the vitamin essential for smooth skin.

Hair

'I'm a wear-my-hair-down kind of woman, but I don't like when it's overstyled, so I stop blow-drying my hair when it's still slightly damp and let it air-dry the rest of the way. It makes it more lived-in and not so perfect. Also, when you don't have products handy, the easiest way to create volume is to backcomb your hair all over, then squeeze the roots with a flatiron to lock in the lift. It works like magic.'

Claudia Schiffer

Something that you will never find top stylists doing when they tend to supermodel hair is towel drying! This is a guaranteed way to add more frizz. Instead, try squeezing hair with your hands, section by section rather than by twisting, then wrapping in an old, clean T-shirt to absorb excess shower water.

Need a super-quick, super-shine rinse idea?
Throw a full model move by following conditioner
with a beer! Pour it over your locks before
washing it out.

Avoid snagging or tearing your hair the backstage way by threading two Kirby grips into a hair bobble, gathering hair into a pony and then digging one grip into the base, wrapping the band around the locks – instead of through – and then securing by digging the second Kirby in next to the first.

If in doubt add texture. It's one of the most common model tricks to pull. All you need is a spritz of sea salt spray and your hands. Add the product then comb through with your fingers, paying particular attention to the roots. Shake back and forth, then wait for the compliments to come rolling in.

Have a model hacial! Catwalk ladies all treat their scalps like their faces, exfoliating, cleansing and treating. Keep an eye out for specialist products, aiming to do one head scrub and one hair mask every week.

'Ponytails are so sexy. It's just a sweet, clean, pretty way for women to wear their hair. It's also really sexy to take it out and shake your hair. Don't be that girl who twirls her hair. If you play with your hair because you think you're looking cute, you're being self-conscious, and that's not sexy anymore.'

Stephanie Seymour

All the styling and travelling means models get really dry hair. In the same boat? Don't stress, simply take your weekly mask treatment to another level by sleeping in it. Once smoothed over your locks, from the midlengths downwards, leaving the roots so they don't get greasy, wrap up in cling flim to help it penetrate further and to save your pillow cases. Wash out in the morning and discover super smoothness.

The easiest way to get natural waves is to carefully wash hair, comb through and then braid into bunches while still damp, securing with a snag-free band before bed. Your locks will dry as you sleep, and upon waking you can gently press straightners over your plaits before releasing to reveal casually beautiful curls. Models are always sneakily doing this.

Even when armed with tongs, wands and straighteners, backstage teams are never without a hairdryer. It's important to blow out hair the model way – from the root first – whatever your styling tool of choice, to stop a look going flat.

'If you have dry hair, don't wash it every day. And if you have very, <u>very</u> dry hair, wash it once a week! The oils help your hair look better. You have to do what's good for <u>your</u> hair.'

Adriana Lima

Sometimes supermodels and stylists have a spare toothbrush about their person. Not as a back-up brush but to gently stroke down stray bits of frizz that escape from slick buns and ponies. For an even more intense smooth down, spritz your toothbrush with a little hairspray first.

Top models love a fish supper. Tuck into salmon, tuna and mackerel as they are full of fatty acids that make hair shine like nothing else.

Any catwalk regular worth her salt knows the difference between shampoos and conditioners. You will always find a model using shampoo on the scalp downwards, while she only uses the conditioner from the midlengths down to prevent any kind of pesky greasiness.

How often do top models wash their hair? Only when they need it – be it once a week or every other day. Create your own bespoke tress routine and stick to it.

'Never put a knot in wet hair —
your strands will break.'

Daphne Groeneveld

Dry shampoo is one of the greatest beauty inventions and our hero when we just don't have time to wash our locks. However, did you know that it actually works better if applied before you go to bed? All the best models are in on the secret, spritzing it on before they put their PJs on ahead of days when they know they'll be super hectic. It also helps you avoid that powdery white look, but it's also worth nabbing a dry shampoo to match your hair colour; more and more are coming onto the market with every season.

No matter how much their schedules spiral models always trim. A split end cull, on long, short or midlengths, is the speediest way to ensure super-slick looking hair.

Make like a model backstage when blow drying. Blast locks until they are about 80 per cent dry, then section off hair and use the dryer to finish the job with a round ceramic brush to prevent breakage, keep things smooth and stop your arms aching too much.

To make sure your catwalk curls stay in all day give each section a light spritz of hairspray both before and after wrapping it around the wand. It helps with hold.

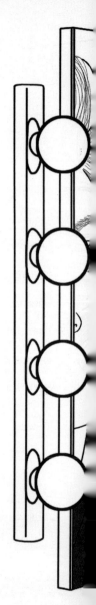

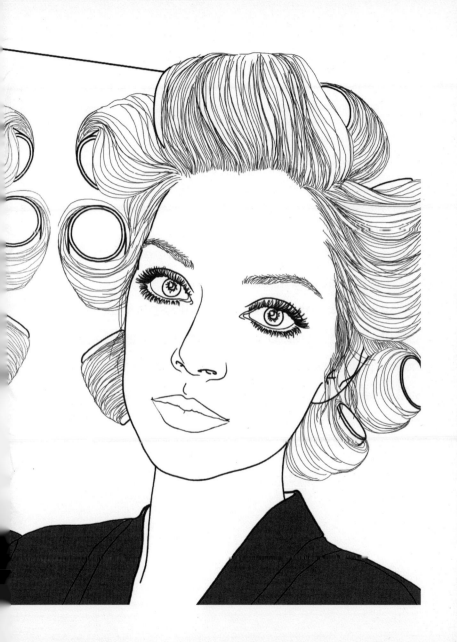

Remember this hair model mantra: when styling hair always respect the cooling-off period. You use dryers, straightners, wands and tongs to create a new shape. The heat allows you to do this. It then needs to go cold to let it set. If you move it around or pull it out a bit while hot you will lose your style. Always do a touch test to make sure it has cooled.

Hair looking a little dry and lifeless? Mash up an avocado with olive oil and smooth it on to the midlengths and ends. Leave out the roots as they can get greasy. The salad favourite is packed with nourishing vitamins and oils, which, when left on locks for 20 minutes, work their magic. Rinse and enjoy your silky locks.

Backcombing is a backstage on-set essential for adding height and volume to model hair and looks cool on all lengths. However, it can be tricky to get out afterwards. To ditch the knots with minimum damage, wash, then add conditioner, combing through while it does its nourishing thing. The product helps ease out the tangles.

Models are forever changing their cuts, styles and colours. They also use cut, style and colour appropriate products. Do the same as you experiment to make every do look runway ready. You wear your hair every day, so invest in it and look after it – it's your best accessory.

Body, Confidence & Lifestyle

'There was a time I walked in a Fendi runway show and made a little slip and slipped off the runway. All you can do is do your best... Even when you make mistakes, sometimes those can be the most important experiences to learn from.'

Karlie Kloss

Treat your body with respect – models do as it's their career. It's yours too. You couldn't do your job without, it right? Just because you're not slinking down the runway, it's still important. Fuel it well, and exercise it at least three times a week.

Make a folder of your favourite pictures – selfies and posing with friends supermodel style – and save it on your phone. Whenever a confidence wobble strikes, flick through them to make you smile!

'I think being comfortable in one's skin is the most attractive quality a girl can have.'

Rosie Huntington-Whiteley

Even supermodels make mistakes. Backstage areas, shoots and campaigns are just a few places anything can happen; sometimes it's magic, sometimes it's meltdown. That's life. Simply style out mishaps like a model and learn from them. It's how you deal with them that counts.

A common sight backstage is a model having her hair, make-up and nails done all at once... it's chaos and super-stressful, which is why so many models also have their earphones in and iPod firmly switched on. Make your own playlist of power songs that will calm, inspire and help you deal with any situation.

'I'm more interested in workouts that make me less stressed because then I can clear my head. So I like yoga and running. I don't have to run far, just for half an hour, and I come back with so many ideas.'

Suki Waterhouse

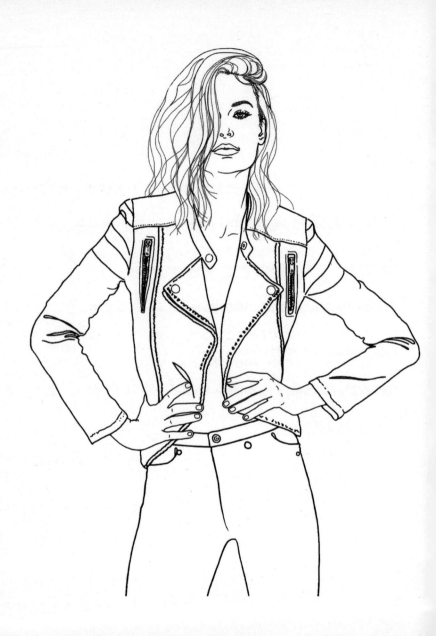

Life is crazy, hectic and fun all at the same time – just ask anyone who models for a living. And things can feel overwhelming, which is why supers practice mindfulness. When something amazing is happening, stop just for a moment and take in what you can see, smell and hear and then enjoy it, before time moves you on to the next thing.

Be kind to yourself. Models are constantly scrutinized as they're selected, or not, for shows, ad campaigns, TV shows, shoots and everything else on their look-good to-do list. They have to shut out the haters, know that not every job is for every model and high five themselves when they've done a good job. This way of thinking applies to everyone.

'If you really want to lose weight, try running intervals outside. I run for 20 minutes — one minute "on" running as fast as you can and then one minute "off" walking and catching your breath. By the time you've done the sixth interval, you won't be going too fast but it's a great way to get in shape.'

Elle Macpherson

Ten deep breaths. It's an easy way to ease a situation, find perspective and get some much needed oxygen to an overloaded brain. Models do it backstage and on set all the time.

Moisturising every bit of your body is the simplest and most effective way of getting a supermodel body. Fact.

'I drink a glass of warm water with the juice of half an organic lemon each morning. Warm lemon water in the morning helps kick-start the digestion process for the rest of the day. It's also a ritual that cleanses the system, boosts your immune system and balances pH levels because lemons are very alkalizing. They are also abundant in vitamin C, which promotes healing and health.'

Miranda Kerr

Models are all about prioritising and balancing work with having fun. Make a list of what you do every day, then make a list of what really makes you happy. Compare the lists and adjust accordingly.

Want long, supermodel-esque legs? Well, who wouldn't?! Slick an oil with added golden sheen down the middle of the thighs and shins. Skip out the knee – not an area anyone wants to draw attention to – but blend the oil in the other areas as it streamlines your legs and makes them look longer.

'I do not have a specific exercise. I love yoga, boxing, Kung Fu, Pilates, surfing, horseback riding, playing volleyball. The important thing is how good I feel after exercising. When I don't feel that my day was incomplete.'

Gisele Bündchen

Tanning has moved on from a faux orange finish that reminds us of a well-known fizzy drink. Instead, gorgeous, caramel-coloured skin that convinces people you've been hanging out in St Tropez for the weekend is a model's go-to tan request. Perfect your pretend tan by mixing two parts instant tan to one part moisturiser and one part highlighter. Scrunch your products into a foam tanning mitt and slick all over.

When applying illuminating moisturisers and fake tan products, sweep them on using a foam mitt, using long sweeping motions from head to toe. Afterwards, buff over all areas to trick people into thinking you've popped away on a sunny break. Supermodels swear by this.

'Embrace your weirdness!'

Cara Delevingne

Off for a spray tan? Make like a model by prepping before you get under the power of that golden gun. Exfoliate, and add moisturiser only to your elbows, knuckles and heels to stop too much colour grabbing in these typically more dry areas.

Had a model-like day of compliments? Snap a picture of your make-up, hair and clothes so you always have it to hand to reference another time when you want to look amazing.

Supermodels always look insanely good while good working out, so splash out on cool exercise clothes that make you feel incredible. Research shows that the hotter you feel the harder you will work.

'My advice to women is eat clean, and work out to stay fit — and have a burger to stay sane.'

Gigi Hadid

When taking selfies make sure you hold the camera or phone from above as the angle is more flattering. On times when others are snapping away for you, get them to stand on a step higher then you or tilt the camera downwards over your head.

Had a faux glow disaster? Dive into a swimming pool ASAP. The chlorine in the pool strips off colour and by doing your best dive everything will hit the water evenly.

'My mum used to say, "You can't have fun all the time," and I used to say, "Why not?" Why the f*** can't I have fun all the time?'

Kate Moss

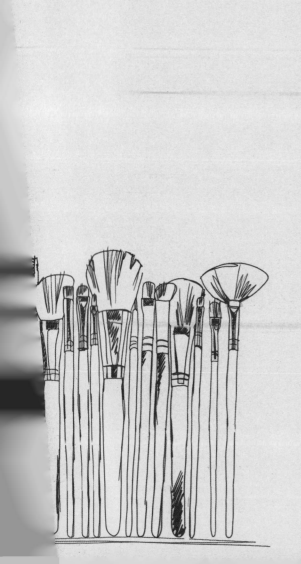

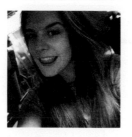

About The Author

Carly Hobbs is a make-up artist, tanner and beauty writer. After styling out life on top glossy magazines like *Fabulous*, *Sugar*, *Heat* and *LOOK*, editing pieces on grooming, health and beauty, she retrained as a make-up artist, tanner and hair stylist. She now works all over the world on editorial, commercial and video shoots, tans celebrity clients and makes the people she meets look like the best versions of themselves. Follow her MUA, tanning and beauty antics on Twitter, Instagram and Snapchat @carlytoptip